CW00569973

Easy Diabetic Meal Prep

Keto Meal Prep cookbook for beginners: for a healthy and carefree life. Quick and easy recipes to cook at home and boost your energy without guilt

TABLE OF CONTENTS

BREAKFAST RECIPES

Balsamic Chicken

Preparation Time: 10 minutes

Cooking Time: 25 minutes

Servings: 6

Ingredients

- 6 chicken breast halves, skinless and boneless

- 1 teaspoon garlic salt

- Ground black pepper

- 2 tablespoons olive oil

- 1 onion, thinly sliced

- 14- and 1/2-ounces tomatoes, diced

- 1/2 cup balsamic vinegar

- 1 teaspoon dried basil

- 1 teaspoon dried oregano

- 1 teaspoon dried rosemary

- 1/2 teaspoon dried thyme

Directions:

1. Season both sides of your chicken breasts thoroughly with pepper and garlic salt

2. Take a skillet and place it over medium heat

3. Add some oil and cook your seasoned chicken for 3-4 minutes per side until the breasts are nicely browned

4. Add some onion and cook for another 3-4 minutes until the onions are browned

5. Pour the diced-up tomatoes and balsamic vinegar over your chicken and season with some rosemary, basil, thyme, and rosemary

6. Simmer the chicken for about 15 minutes until they are no longer pink

7. Take an instant-read thermometer and check if the internal temperature gives a reading of 165 degrees Fahrenheit

8. If yes, then you are good to go!

Nutrition: Calories: 196 Fat: 7g Carbohydrates: 7g Protein: 23g

Greek Chicken Breast

Preparation Time: 10 minutes

Cooking Time: 25 minutes

Servings: 4

Ingredients

- 4 chicken breast halves, skinless and boneless
- 1 cup extra virgin olive oil
- 1 lemon, juiced
- 2 teaspoons garlic, crushed
- 1 and 1/2 teaspoons black pepper
- 1/3 teaspoon paprika

Directions:

1. Cut 3 slits in the chicken breast
2. Take a small bowl and whisk in olive oil, salt, lemon juice, garlic, paprika, pepper and whisk for 30 seconds
3. Place chicken in a large bowl and pour marinade

4. Rub the marinade all over using your hand

5. Refrigerate overnight

6. Pre-heat grill to medium heat and oil the grate

7. Cook chicken in the grill until center is no longer pink

8. Serve and enjoy!

Nutrition: Calories: 644 Fat: 57g Carbohydrates: 2g Protein: 27g

Chipotle Lettuce Chicken

Preparation Time: 10 minutes

Cooking Time: 25 minutes

Servings: 6

Ingredients

- 1 pound chicken breast, cut into strips

- Splash of olive oil

- 1 red onion, finely sliced

- 14 ounces tomatoes

- 1 teaspoon chipotle, chopped

- 1/2 teaspoon cumin

- Pinch of sugar

- Lettuce as needed

- Fresh coriander leaves

- Jalapeno chilies, sliced

- Fresh tomato slices for garnish

- Lime wedges

Directions:

1. Take a non-stick frying pan and place it over medium heat
2. Add oil and heat it up
3. Add chicken and cook until brown
4. Keep the chicken on the side
5. Add tomatoes, sugar, chipotle, cumin to the same pan and simmer for 25 minutes until you have a nice sauce
6. Add chicken into the sauce and cook for 5 minutes
7. Transfer the mix to another place
8. Use lettuce wraps to take a portion of the mixture and serve with a squeeze of lemon
9. Enjoy!

Nutrition: Calories: 332 Fat: 15g Carbohydrates: 13g Protein: 34g

Stylish Chicken-Bacon Wrap

Preparation Time: 5 minutes

Cooking Time: 50 minutes

Servings: 3

Ingredients

- 8 ounces lean chicken breast

- 6 bacon slices

- 3 ounces shredded cheese

- 4 slices ham

Directions:

1. Cut chicken breast into bite-sized portions

2. Transfer shredded cheese onto ham slices

3. Roll up chicken breast and ham slices in bacon slices

4. Take a skillet and place it over medium heat

5. Add olive oil and brown bacon for a while

6. Remove rolls and transfer to your oven

7. Bake for 45 minutes at 325 degrees F

8. Serve and enjoy!

Nutrition: Calories: 275 Fat: 11g Carbohydrates: 0.5g Protein: 40g

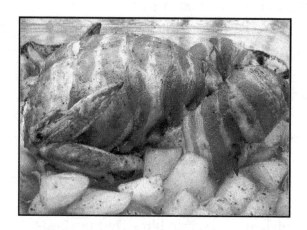

APPETIZER RECIPES

Tomato Toasts

Preparation time: 5 minutes

Cooking time: 5 minutes

Servings: 4

Ingredients:

- 4 slices of sprouted bread toasts

- 2 tomatoes, sliced

- 1 avocado, mashed

- 1 teaspoon olive oil

- 1 pinch of salt

- ¾ teaspoon ground black pepper

Directions:

1. Blend together the olive oil, mashed avocado, salt, and ground black pepper.

2. When the mixture is homogenous – spread it over the sprouted bread.

3. Then place the sliced tomatoes over the toasts.

4. Enjoy!

Nutrition: Calories: 125 Fat: 11.1g Carbohydrates: 7.0g Protein: 1.5g

Everyday Salad

Preparation time: 10 minutes

Cooking time: 40 minutes

Servings: 6

Ingredients:

- 5 halved mushrooms

- 6 halved Cherry (Plum) Tomatoes

- 6 rinsed Lettuce Leaves

- 10 olives

- ½ chopped cucumber

- Juice from ½ Key Lime

- 1 teaspoon olive oil

- Pure Sea Salt

Directions:

1. Tear rinsed lettuce leaves into medium pieces and put them in a medium salad bowl.

2. Add mushrooms halves, chopped cucumber, olives and cherry tomato halves into the bowl. Mix well. Pour olive and Key Lime juice over salad.

3. Add pure sea salt to taste. Mix it all till it is well combined.

Nutrition: Calories: 88 Carbohydrates: 11g Fat: .5g Protein: .8g

Super-Seedy Salad with Tahini Dressing

Preparation time: 10 minutes

Cooking time: 0 minutes

Servings: 1-2

Ingredients:

- 1 slice stale sourdough, torn into chunks

- 50g mixed seeds

- 1 tsp. cumin seeds

- 1 tsp. coriander seeds

- 50g baby kale

- 75g long-stemmed broccoli, blanched for a few minutes then roughly chopped

- ½ red onion, thinly sliced

- 100g cherry tomatoes, halved

- ½ a small bunch flat-leaf parsley, torn

DRESSING

- 100ml natural yogurt

- 1 tbsp. tahini

- 1 lemon, juiced

Directions:

1. Heat the oven to 200°C/fan 180°C/gas 6. Put the bread into a food processor and pulse into very rough breadcrumbs. Put into a bowl with the mixed seeds and spices, season, and spray well with oil. Tip onto a non-stick baking tray and roast for 15-20 minutes, stirring and tossing regularly, until deep golden brown.

2. Whisk together the dressing **Ingredients**, some seasoning and a splash of water in a large bowl. Tip the baby kale, broccoli, red onion, cherry tomatoes and flat-leaf parsley into the dressing, and mix well. Divide between 2 plates and top with the crispy breadcrumbs and seeds.

Nutrition: Calories: 78 Carbohydrates: 6 g Fat: 2g Protein: 1.5g

Vegetable Salad

Preparation time: 10 minutes

Cooking time: 0 minutes

Servings: 1-2

Ingredients:

- 4 cups each of raw spinach and romaine lettuce

- 2 cups each of cherry tomatoes, sliced cucumber, chopped baby carrots and chopped red, orange and yellow bell pepper

- 1 cup each of chopped broccoli, sliced yellow squash, zucchini and cauliflower.

Directions:

1. Wash all these vegetables.

2. Mix in a large mixing bowl and top off with a non-fat or low-fat dressing of your choice.

Nutrition: Calories: 48 Carbohydrates: 11g Protein: 3g

Greek Salad

Preparation time: 10 minutes

Cooking time: 0 minutes

Servings: 1-2

Ingredients:

- 1 Romaine head, torn in bits

- 1 cucumber sliced

- 1 pint cherry tomatoes, halved

- 1 green pepper, thinly sliced

- 1 onion sliced into rings

- 1 cup kalamata olives

- 1 ½ cups feta cheese, crumbled

- For dressing combine:

- 1 cup olive oil

- 1/4 cup lemon juice

- 2 tsp. oregano

- Salt and pepper

Directions:

1. Lay Ingredients on plate.

2. Drizzle dressing over salad

Nutrition: Calories: 107 Carbohydrates: 18g Fat: 1.2 g Protein: 1g

FIRST COURSE RECIPES

Green Salad with Blackberries, Goat Cheese, and Sweet Potatoes

Preparation Time: 15 minutes

Cooking Time: 20 minutes

Serving: 4

Ingredients:

For the vinaigrette

- 1-pint blackberries

- 2 tablespoons red wine vinegar

- 1 tablespoon honey

- 3 tablespoons extra-virgin olive oil

- ¼ teaspoon salt

- Freshly ground black pepper

For the salad

- 1 sweet potato, cubed

- 1 teaspoon extra-virgin olive oil

- 8 cups salad greens (baby spinach, spicy greens, romaine)

- ½ red onion, sliced

- ¼ cup crumbled goat cheese

Direction:

For vinaigrette

1. In a blender jar, combine the blackberries, vinegar, honey, oil, salt, and pepper, and process until smooth. Set aside.

For salad

2. Preheat the oven to 425°F. Line a baking sheet with parchment paper.

3. Mix the sweet potato with the olive oil. Transfer to the prepared baking sheet and roast for 20 minutes, stirring once halfway through, until tender. Remove and cool for a few minutes.

4. In a large bowl, toss the greens with the red onion and cooled sweet potato, and drizzle with the vinaigrette.

Serve topped with 1 tablespoon of goat cheese per serving.

Nutrition: 196 Calories 21g Carbohydrates 10g Sugars

Three Bean and Basil Salad

Preparation Time: 10 minutes

Cooking Time: 0 minute

Serving: 8

Ingredients:

- 1 (15-ounce) can low-sodium chickpeas

- 1 (15-ounce) can low-sodium kidney beans

- 1 (15-ounce) can low-sodium white beans

- 1 red bell pepper

- ¼ cup chopped scallions

- ¼ cup finely chopped fresh basil

- 3 garlic cloves, minced

- 2 tablespoons extra-virgin olive oil

- 1 tablespoon red wine vinegar

- 1 teaspoon Dijon mustard

- ¼ teaspoon freshly ground black pepper

Direction:

1. Toss chickpeas, kidney beans, white beans, bell pepper, scallions, basil, and garlic gently.

2. Blend together olive oil, vinegar, mustard, and pepper. Toss with the salad.

3. Wrap and chill for 1 hour.

Nutrition: 193 Calories 29g Carbohydrates 3g Sugars

Rainbow Black Bean Salad

Preparation Time: 15 minutes

Cooking Time: 0 minute

Serving: 5

Ingredients:

- 1 (15-ounce) can low-sodium black beans

- 1 avocado, diced

- 1 cup cherry

- tomatoes, halved

- 1 cup chopped baby spinach

- ½ cup red bell pepper

- ¼ cup jicama

- ½ cup scallions

- ¼ cup fresh cilantro

- 2 tablespoons lime juice

- 1 tablespoon extra-virgin olive oil

- 2 garlic cloves, minced

- 1 teaspoon honey

- ¼ teaspoon salt

- ¼ teaspoon freshly ground black pepper

Direction:

1. Mix black beans, avocado, tomatoes, spinach, bell pepper, jicama, scallions, and cilantro.

2. Blend lime juice, oil, garlic, honey, salt, and pepper. Add to the salad and toss.

3. Chill for 1 hour before serving.

Nutrition: 169 Calories 22g Carbohydrates 3g Sugars

SECOND COURSE RECIPES

Braised Shrimp

Preparation Time: 10 minutes

Cooking Time: 4 Minutes

Servings: 4

Ingredients:

- 1-pound frozen large shrimp, peeled and deveined

- 2 shallots, chopped

- ¾ cup low-sodium chicken broth

- 2 tablespoons fresh lemon juice

- 2 tablespoons olive oil

- 1 tablespoon garlic, crushed

- Ground black pepper, as required

Directions:

1. In the Instant Pot, place oil and press "Sauté". Now add the shallots and cook for about 2 minutes.

2. Add the garlic and cook for about 1 minute.

3. Press "Cancel" and stir in the shrimp, broth, lemon juice and black pepper.

4. Close the lid and place the pressure valve to "Seal" position.

5. Press "Manual" and cook under "High Pressure" for about 1 minute.

6. Press "Cancel" and carefully allow a "Quick" release.

7. Open the lid and serve hot.

Nutrition: Calories: 209, Fats: 9g, Carbs: 4.3g, Sugar: 0.2g, Proteins: 26.6g, Sodium: 293mg

Shrimp Coconut Curry

Preparation Time: 10 minutes

Cooking Time: 20 Minutes

Servings: 2

Ingredients:

- 0.5lb cooked shrimp

- 1 thinly sliced onion

- 1 cup coconut yogurt

- 3tbsp curry paste

- 1tbsp oil or ghee

Directions:

1. Set the Instant Pot to sauté and add the onion, oil, and curry paste.

2. When the onion is soft, add the remaining ingredients and seal.

3. Cook on Stew for 20 minutes.

4. Release the pressure naturally.

Nutrition: Calories: 380; Carbs: 13; Sugar: 4; Fat: 22; Protein: 40; GL: 14

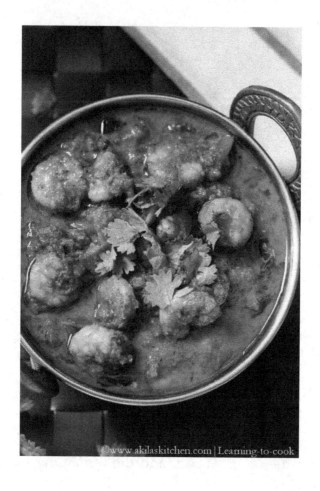

Trout Bake

Preparation Time: 10 minutes

Cooking Time: 35 Minutes

Servings: 2

Ingredients:

- 1lb trout fillets, boneless

- 1lb chopped winter vegetables

- 1 cup low sodium fish broth

- 1tbsp mixed herbs

- sea salt as desired

Directions:

1. Mix all the ingredients except the broth in a foil pouch.

2. Place the pouch in the steamer basket your Instant Pot.

3. Pour the broth into the Instant Pot.

4. Cook on Steam for 35 minutes.

5. Release the pressure naturally.

Nutrition: Calories: 310; Carbs: 14; Sugar: 2; Fat: 12; Protein: 40; GL: 5

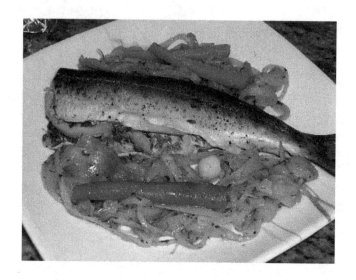

Sardine Curry

Preparation Time: 10 minutes

Cooking Time: 35 Minutes

Servings: 2

Ingredients:

- 5 tins of sardines in tomato

- 1lb chopped vegetables

- 1 cup low sodium fish broth

- 3tbsp curry paste

Directions:

1. Mix all the ingredients in your Instant Pot.

2. Cook on Stew for 35 minutes.

3. Release the pressure naturally.

Nutrition: Calories: 320; Carbs: 8; Sugar: 2; Fat: 16; Protein: GL: 3

Swordfish Steak

Preparation Time: 10 minutes

Cooking Time: 35 Minutes

Servings: 2

Ingredients:

- 1lb swordfish steak, whole

- 1lb chopped Mediterranean vegetables

- 1 cup low sodium fish broth

- 2tbsp soy sauce

Directions:

1. Mix all the ingredients except the broth in a foil pouch.

2. Place the pouch in the steamer basket for your Instant Pot.

3. Pour the broth into the Instant Pot. Lower the steamer basket into the Instant Pot.

4. Cook on Steam for 35 minutes.

5. Release the pressure naturally.

Nutrition: Calories: 270; Carbs: 5; Sugar: 1; Fat: 10; Protein: 48; GL: 1

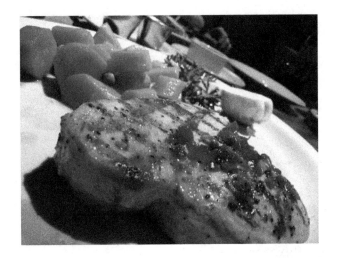

SIDE DISH RECIPES

Pumpkin Spice Crackers

Preparation time: 10 minutes

Cooking time: 60 minutes

Servings: 06

Ingredients:

- 1/3 cup coconut flour

- 2 tablespoons pumpkin pie spice

- ¾ cup sunflower seeds

- ¾ cup flaxseed

- 1/3 cup sesame seeds

- 1 tablespoon ground psyllium husk powder

- 1 teaspoon sea salt

- 3 tablespoons coconut oil, melted

- 11/3 cups alkaline water

Directions:

1. Set your oven to 300 degrees F.

2. Combine all dry **Ingredients** in a bowl.

3. Add water and oil to the mixture and mix well.

4. Let the dough stay for 2 to 3 minutes.

5. Spread the dough evenly on a cookie sheet lined with parchment paper.

6. Bake for 30 minutes.

7. Reduce the oven heat to low and bake for another 30 minutes.

8. Crack the bread into bite-size pieces.

9. Serve

Nutrition: Calories 248 Total Fat 15.7 g Saturated Fat 2.7 g Cholesterol 75 mg Sodium 94 mg Total Carbs 0.4 g Fiber 0g Sugar 0 g Protein 24.9 g

Spicy Roasted Nuts

Preparation time: 10 minutes

Cooking time: 15 minutes

Servings: 4

Ingredients:

- 8 oz. pecans or almonds or walnuts

- 1 teaspoon sea salt

- 1 tablespoon olive oil or coconut oil

- 1 teaspoon ground cumin

- 1 teaspoon paprika powder or chili powder

Directions:

1. Add all the **Ingredients** to a skillet.

2. Roast the nuts until golden brown.

3. Serve and enjoy.

Nutrition: Calories 287 Total Fat 29.5 g Saturated Fat 3 g Cholesterol 0 mg Total Carbs 5.9 g Sugar 1.4g

Fiber 4.3 g Sodium 388 mg Protein 4.2 g

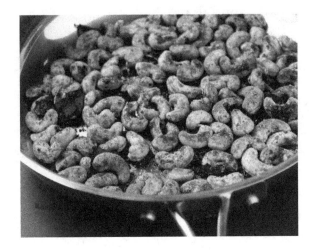

Wheat Crackers

Preparation time: 10 minutes

Cooking time: 20 minutes

Servings: 4

Ingredients:

- 1 3/4 cups almond flour

- 1 1/2 cups coconut flour

- 3/4 teaspoon sea salt

- 1/3 cup vegetable oil

- 1 cup alkaline water

- Sea salt for sprinkling

Directions:

1. Set your oven to 350 degrees F.

2. Mix coconut flour, almond flour and salt in a bowl.

3. Stir in vegetable oil and water. Mix well until smooth.

4. Spread this dough on a floured surface into a thin sheet.

5. Cut small squares out of this sheet.

6. Arrange the dough squares on a baking sheet lined with parchment paper.

7. For about 20 minutes, bake until light golden in color.

8. Serve.

Nutrition: Calories 64 Total Fat 9.2 g Saturated Fat 2.4 g Cholesterol 110 mg Sodium 276 m Total Carbs 9.2 g Fiber 0.9 g Sugar 1.4 g Protein 1.5 g

Potato Chips

Preparation time: 10 minutes

Cooking time: 20 minutes

Servings: 4

Ingredients:

- 1 tablespoon vegetable oil

- 1 potato, sliced paper thin

- Sea salt, to taste

Directions:

1. Toss potato with oil and sea salt.

2. Spread the slices in a baking dish in a single layer.

3. Cook in a microwave for 5 minutes until golden brown.

4. Serve.

Nutrition: Calories 80 Total Fat 3.5 g Saturated Fat 0.1 g Cholesterol 320 mg Sodium 350 mg Total Carbs 11.6 g Fiber 0.7 g Sugar 0.7 g Protein 1.2 g

SOUP & STEW

Spicy Carrot Soup

Preparation time: 10 minutes

Cooking time: 20 minutes

Servings: 6

Ingredients:

- 8 large carrots, peeled and chopped

- 1 1/2 cups filtered alkaline water

- 14 oz. coconut milk

- 3 garlic cloves, peeled

- 1 tbsp. red curry paste

- 1/4 cup olive oil

- 1 onion, chopped

- Salt

Directions:

1. Combine all elements into the direct pot and mix fine.

2. Cover pot with lid and select manual and set timer for 15 minutes.

3. Allow to release pressure naturally then open the lid.

4. Blend the soup utilizing a submersion blender until smooth.

5. Serve and enjoy.

Nutrition: Calories 267 Fat 22 g Carbohydrates 13 g Protein 4 g Sugar 5 g Cholesterol 20 mg

Zucchini Soup

Preparation time: 10 minutes

Cooking time: 30 minutes

Servings: 10

Ingredients:

- 10 cups zucchini, chopped

- 32 oz. filtered alkaline water

- 13.5 oz. coconut milk

- 1 tbsp. Thai curry paste

Directions:

1. Combine all elements into the direct pot and mix fine.

2. Cover pot with lid and cook on manual high pressure for 10 minutes.

3. Release pressure using quick release **Directions**: than open the lid.

4. Using blender Blend the soup until smooth.

5. Serve and enjoy.

Nutrition: Calories 122 Fat 9.8 g Carbohydrates 6.6 g Protein 4.1 g Sugar 3.6 g Cholesterol 0 mg

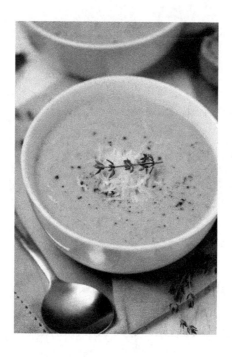

Kidney Bean Stew

Preparation time: 15 minutes

Cooking time: 15 minutes

Servings: 2

Ingredients:

- 1lb cooked kidney beans

- 1 cup tomato passata

- 1 cup low sodium beef broth

- 3tbsp Italian herbs

Directions:

1. Mix all the ingredients in your Instant Pot.

2. Cook on Stew for 15 minutes.

3. Release the pressure naturally.

Nutrition: Calories: 270 Carbs: 16 Sugar: 3 Fat: 10 Protein: 23 GL: 8

Cabbage Soup

Preparation time: 15 minutes

Cooking time: 35 minutes

Servings: 2

Ingredients:

- 1lb shredded cabbage

- 1 cup low sodium vegetable broth

- 1 shredded onion

- 2tbsp mixed herbs

- 1tbsp black pepper

Directions:

1. Mix all the ingredients in your Instant Pot.

2. Cook on Stew for 35 minutes.

3. Release the pressure naturally.

Nutrition: Calories: 60 Carbs: 2 Sugar: 0 Fat: 2 Protein: 4 GL: 1

Pumpkin Spice Soup

Preparation time: 10 minutes

Cooking time: 35 minutes

Servings: 2

Ingredients:

- 1lb cubed pumpkin

- 1 cup low sodium vegetable broth

- 2tbsp mixed spice

Directions:

1. Mix all the ingredients in your Instant Pot.

2. Cook on Stew for 35 minutes.

3. Release the pressure naturally.

4. Blend the soup.

Nutrition: Calories: 100 Carbs: 7 Sugar: 1 Fat: 2 Protein: 3 GL: 1

DESSERT

Raspberry Cream Cheese Coffee Cake

Preparation Time: 10 minutes

Cooking time: 4 hours

Servings: 12

Ingredients

- 1 1/4 almond flour

- 2/3 cup water

- 1/2 cup Swerve

- 3 eggs

- 1/4 cup coconut flour

- 1/4 cup protein powder

- 1/4 teaspoon salt

- 1/2 teaspoon vanilla extract

- 1 1/2 teaspoon baking powder

- 6 tablespoons butter, melted

For the Filling:

- 1 1/2 cup fresh raspberries

- 8 oz. cream cheese

- 1 large egg

- 1/3 cup powdered Swerve

- 2 tablespoon whipping cream

Directions:

1. Grease the slow cooker pot. Prepare the cake batter. In a bowl, combine almond flour together with coconut flour, sweetener, baking powder, protein powder and salt, and then stir in the melted butter along with eggs and water until well combined. Set aside.

2. Prepare the filling. Beat cream cheese thoroughly with the sweetener until have smoothened, and then beat in whipping cream along with the egg and vanilla extract until well combined.

3. Assemble the cake. Spread around 2/3 of batter in the slow cooker as you smoothen the top using a spatula or knife.

4. Pour cream cheese mixture over the batter in the pan, evenly spread it, and then sprinkle with raspberries. Add the rest of batter over filling.

5. Cook for 3-4 hours on low. Let cool completely.

6. Serve and enjoy!

Nutrition: 239 calories; 19.18 g fat; 6.9 g total carbs; 7.5 g protein

Pumpkin Pie Bars

Preparation Time: 10 minutes

Cooking time: 3 hours

Servings: 16

Ingredients

For the Crust:

- 3/4 cup coconut, shredded

- 4 tablespoons butter, unsalted, softened

- 1/4 cup cocoa powder, unsweetened

- 1/4 teaspoon salt

- 1/2 cup raw sunflower seeds or sunflower seed flour

- 1/4 cup confectioners Swerve

Filling:

- 2 teaspoons cinnamon liquid stevia

- 1 cup heavy cream

- 1 can pumpkin puree

- 6 eggs

- 1 tablespoon pumpkin pie spice

- 1/2 teaspoon salt

- 1 tablespoon vanilla extract

- 1/2 cup sugar-free chocolate chips, optional

Directions:

1. Add all the crust ingredients to a food processor. Then process until fine crumbs are formed.

2. Grease the slow cooker pan well. When done, press crust mixture onto the greased bottom.

3. In a stand mixer, combine all the ingredients for the filling, and then blend well until combined.

4. Top the filling with chocolate chips if using, and then pour the mixture onto the prepared crust.

5. Close the lid and cook for 3 hours on low. Open the lid and let cool for at least 30 minutes, and then place the slow cooker into the refrigerator for at least 3 hours.

6. Slice the pumpkin pie bar and serve it with sugar free whipped cream. Enjoy!

Nutrition: 169 calories; 15 g fat; 6 g total carbs; 4 g protein

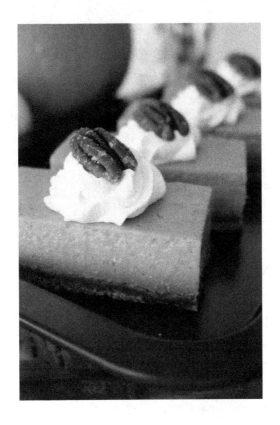

Dark Chocolate Cake

Preparation Time: 10 minutes

Cooking time: 3 hours

Servings: 10

Ingredients

- 1 cup almond flour

- 3 eggs

- 2 tablespoons almond flour

- 1/4 teaspoon salt

- 1/2 cup Swerve Granular

- 3/4 teaspoon vanilla extract

- 2/3 cup almond milk, unsweetened

- 1/2 cup cocoa powder

- 6 tablespoons butter, melted

- 1 1/2 teaspoon baking powder

- 3 tablespoons unflavored whey protein powder or egg white protein powder

- 1/3 cup sugar-free chocolate chips, optional

Directions:

1. Grease the slow cooker well.
2. Whisk the almond flour together with cocoa powder, sweetener, whey protein powder, salt and baking powder in a bowl. Then stir in butter along with almond milk, eggs and the vanilla extract until well combined, and then stir in the chocolate chips if desired.
3. When done, pour into the slow cooker. Allow to cook for 2-2 1/2 hours on low.
4. When through, turn off the slow cooker and let the cake cool for about 20-30 minutes.
5. When cooled, cut the cake into pieces and serve warm with lightly sweetened whipped cream. Enjoy!

Nutrition: 205 calories; 17 g fat; 8.4 g total carbs; 12 g protein

Lemon Custard

Preparation Time: 10 minutes

Cooking time: 3 hours

Servings: 4

Ingredients:

- 2 cups whipping cream or coconut cream

- 5 egg yolks

- 1 tablespoon lemon zest

- 1 teaspoon vanilla extract

- 1/4 cup fresh lemon juice, squeezed

- 1/2 teaspoon liquid stevia

- Lightly sweetened whipped cream

Directions:

1. Whisk egg yolks together with lemon zest, liquid stevia, lemon zest and vanilla in a bowl, and then whisk in heavy cream.

2. Divide the mixture among 4 small jars or ramekins.

3. To the bottom of a slow cooker add a rack, and then add ramekins on top of the rack and add enough water to cover half of ramekins.

4. Close the lid and cook for 3 hours on low. Remove ramekins.

5. Let cool to room temperature, and then place into the refrigerator to cool completely for about 3 hours.

6. When through, top with the whipped cream and serve. Enjoy!

Nutrition: 319 calories; 30 g fat; 3 g total carbs; 7 g protein

Baked Stuffed Pears

Preparation time: 15 minutes

Cooking time: 35 minutes

Servings: 04

Ingredients:

- Agave syrup, 4 tbsp.

- Cloves, .25 tsp.

- Chopped walnuts, 4 tbsp.

- Currants, 1 c

- Pears, 4

Directions:

1. Make sure your oven has been warmed to 375.

2. Slice the pears in two lengthwise and remove the core. To get the pear to lay flat, you can slice a small piece off the back side.

3. Place the agave syrup, currants, walnuts, and cloves in a small bowl and mix well. Set this to the side to be used later.

4. Put the pears on a cookie sheet that has parchment paper on it. Make sure the cored sides are facing up. Sprinkle each pear half with about .5 tablespoon of the chopped walnut mixture.

5. Place into the oven and cook for 25 to 30 minutes. Pears should be tender.

Nutrition: Calories: 103.9 Fiber: 3.1 g Carbohydrates: 22 g

Butternut Squash Pie

Preparation time: 25 minutes

Cooking time: 35 minutes

Servings: 04

Ingredients:

- For the Crust

- Cold water

- Agave, splash

- Sea salt, pinch

- Grapeseed oil, .5 c

- Coconut flour, .5 c

- Spelt Flour, 1 c

- For the Filling

- Butternut squash, peeled, chopped

- Water

- Allspice, to taste

- Agave syrup, to taste

- Hemp milk, 1 c

- Sea moss, 4 tbsp.

Directions:

1. You will need to warm your oven to 350.

2. For the Crust

3. Place the grapeseed oil and water into the refrigerator to get it cold. This will take about one hour.

4. Place all **Ingredients** into a large bowl. Now you need to add in the cold water a little bit in small amounts until a dough form. Place this onto a surface that has been sprinkled with some coconut flour. Knead for a few minutes and roll the dough as thin as you can get it. Carefully, pick it up and place it inside a pie plate.

5. Place the butternut squash into a Dutch oven and pour in enough water to cover. Bring this to a full rolling boil. Let this cook until the squash has become soft.

6. Completely drain and place into bowl. Using a potato masher, mash the squash. Add in some allspice and agave to taste. Add in the sea moss and hemp milk. Using a hand mixer, blend well. Pour into the pie crust.

7. Place into an oven and bake for about one hour.

Nutrition: Calories: 245 Carbohydrates: 50 g Fat: 10 g

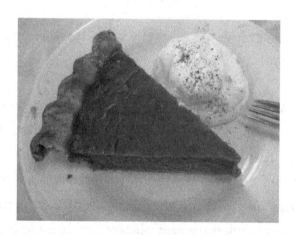

Coconut Chia Cream Pot

Preparation time: 5 minutes

Cooking time: 5 minutes

Servings: 04

Ingredients:

- Date, one (1)

- Coconut milk (organic), one (1) cup

- Coconut yogurt, one (1) cup

- Vanilla extract, ½ teaspoon

- Chia seeds, ¼ cup

- Sesame seeds, one (1) teaspoon

- Flaxseed (ground), one (1) tablespoon or flax meal, one (1) tablespoon

- Toppings:

- Fig, one (1)

- Blueberries, one (1) handful

- Mixed nuts (brazil nuts, almonds, pistachios, macadamia, etc.)

- Cinnamon (ground), one teaspoon

Directions:

1. First, blend the date with coconut milk (the idea is to sweeten the coconut milk).

2. Get a mixing bowl and add the coconut milk with the vanilla, sesame seeds, chia seeds, and flax meal.

3. Refrigerate for between twenty to thirty minutes or wait till the chia expands.

4. To serve, pour a layer of coconut yogurt in a small glass, then add the chia mix, followed by pouring another layer of the coconut yogurt.

5. It's alkaline, creamy and delicious.

Nutrition: Calories: 310 Carbohydrates: 39 g Protein: 4 g Fiber: 8.1 g

Chocolate Avocado Mousse

Preparation time: 10 minutes

Cooking time: 5 minutes

Servings: 04

Ingredients:

- Coconut water, 2/3 cup

- Avocado, ½ hass

- Raw cacao, 2 teaspoons

- Vanilla, 1 teaspoon

- Dates, three (3)

- Sea salt, 0ne (1) teaspoon

- Dark chocolate shavings

Directions:

1. Blend all **Ingredients**.

2. Blast until it becomes thick and smooth, as you wish.

3. Put in a fridge and allow it to get firm.

Nutrition: Calories: 181.8 Fat: 151. G Protein: 12 g

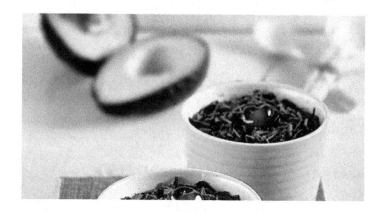

JUICE AND SMOOTHIE RECIPES

Banana Smoothie

Preparation Time: 10 minutes

Cooking Time: 0 minutes

Servings: 2

Ingredients:

- 2 cups chilled unsweetened almond milk

- 1 large frozen banana, peeled and sliced

- 1 tablespoon almonds, chopped

- 1 teaspoon organic vanilla extract

Directions:

1. Place all the ingredients in a high-speed blender and pulse until creamy.

2. Pour the smoothie into two glasses and serve immediately.

Nutrition: Calories 124 Total Fat 5.2 g Saturated Fat 0.5 g Cholesterol 0 mg Sodium 181 mg Total Carbs 18.4 g Fiber 3.1 g Sugar 8.7 g Protein 2.4 g

Strawberry Smoothie

Preparation Time: 10 minutes

Cooking Time: 0 minutes

Servings: 2

Ingredients:

- 2 cups chilled unsweetened almond milk

- 1½ cups frozen strawberries

- 1 banana, peeled and sliced

- ¼ teaspoon organic vanilla extract

Directions:

1. Add all the ingredients in a high-speed blender and pulse until smooth.

2. Pour the smoothie into two glasses and serve immediately.

Nutrition: Calories 131 Total Fat 3.7 g Saturated Fat 0.4 g Cholesterol 0 mg Sodium 181 mg Total Carbs 25.3 g Fiber 4.8 g Sugar 14 g Protein 1.6 g

Raspberry & Tofu Smoothie

Preparation Time: 15 minutes

Cooking Time: 0 minutes

Servings: 2

Ingredients:

- 1½ cups fresh raspberries

- 6 ounces firm silken tofu, drained

- 1/8 teaspoon coconut extract

- 1 teaspoon powdered stevia

- 1½ cups unsweetened almond milk

- ¼ cup ice cubes, crushed

Directions:

1. Add all the ingredients in a high-speed blender and pulse until smooth.

2. Pour the smoothie into two glasses and serve immediately.

Nutrition: Calories 131 Total Fat 5.5 g Saturated Fat 0.6 g Cholesterol 0 mg Sodium 167 mg Total Carbs 14.6 g Fiber 6.8 g Sugar 5.2 g Protein 7.7 g

Mango Smoothie

Preparation Time: 10 minutes

Cooking Time: 0 minutes

Servings: 2

Ingredients:

- 2 cups frozen mango, peeled, pitted and chopped

- ¼ cup almond butter

- Pinch of ground turmeric

- 2 tablespoons fresh lemon juice

- 1¼ cups unsweetened almond milk

- ¼ cup ice cubes

Directions:

1. Add all the ingredients in a high-speed blender and pulse until smooth.

2. Pour the smoothie into two glasses and serve immediately.

Nutrition: Calories 140 Total Fat 4.1 g Saturated Fat 0.6 g Cholesterol 0 mg Sodium 118 mg Total Carbs 26.8 g Fiber 3.6 g Sugar 23 g Protein 2.5 g

Pineapple Smoothie

Preparation Time: 10 minutes

Cooking Time: 0 minutes

Servings: 2

Ingredients:

- 2 cups pineapple, chopped

- ½ teaspoon fresh ginger, peeled and chopped

- ½ teaspoon ground turmeric

- 1 teaspoon natural immune support supplement *

- 1 teaspoon chia seeds

- 1½ cups cold green tea

- ½ cup ice, crushed

Directions:

1. Add all the ingredients in a high-speed blender and pulse until smooth.

2. Pour the smoothie into two glasses and serve immediately.

Nutrition: Calories 152 Total Fat 1 g Saturated Fat 0 g Cholesterol 0 mg Sodium 9 mg Total Carbs 30 g Fiber 3.5 g Sugar 29.8 g Protein 1.5 g

Kale & Pineapple Smoothie

Preparation Time: 15 minutes

Cooking Time: 0 minutes

Servings: 2

Ingredients:

- 1½ cups fresh kale, trimmed and chopped

- 1 frozen banana, peeled and chopped

- ½ cup fresh pineapple chunks

- 1 cup unsweetened coconut milk

- ½ cup fresh orange juice

- ½ cup ice

Directions:

1. Add all the ingredients in a high-speed blender and pulse until smooth.

2. Pour the smoothie into two glasses and serve immediately.

Nutrition: Calories 148 Total Fat 2.4 g Saturated Fat 2.1 g Cholesterol 0 mg Sodium 23 mg Total Carbs 31.6 g Fiber 3.5 g Sugar 16.5 g Protein 2.8 g

Green Veggies Smoothie

Preparation Time: 15 minutes

Cooking Time: 0 minutes

Servings: 2

Ingredients:

- 1 medium avocado, peeled, pitted, and chopped

- 1 large cucumber, peeled and chopped

- 2 fresh tomatoes, chopped

- 1 small green bell pepper, seeded and chopped

- 1 cup fresh spinach, torn

- 2 tablespoons fresh lime juice

- 2 tablespoons homemade vegetable broth

- 1 cup alkaline water

Directions:

1. Add all the ingredients in a high-speed blender and pulse until smooth.

2. Pour the smoothie into glasses and serve immediately.

Nutrition: Calories 275 Total Fat 20.3 g Saturated Fat 4.2 g Cholesterol 0 mg Sodium 76 mg Total Carbs 24.1 g Fiber 10.1 g Sugar 9.3 g Protein 5.3 g

Avocado & Spinach Smoothie

Preparation Time: 10 minutes

Cooking Time: 0 minutes

Servings: 2

Ingredients:

- 2 cups fresh baby spinach

- ½ avocado, peeled, pitted, and chopped

- 4-6 drops liquid stevia

- ½ teaspoon ground cinnamon

- 1 tablespoon hemp seeds

- 2 cups chilled alkaline water

Directions:

1. Add all the ingredients in a high-speed blender and pulse until smooth.

2. Pour the smoothie into two glasses and serve immediately.

Nutrition: Calories 132 Total Fat 11.7 g Saturated Fat 2.2 g Cholesterol 0 mg Sodium 27 mg Total Carbs 6.1 g Fiber 4.5 g Sugar 0.4 g Protein 3.1 g

Raisins – Plume Smoothie (RPS)

Preparation time: 10 minutes

Cooking time: 0 minutes

Servings: 1

Ingredients:

- 1 Teaspoon Raisins

- 2 Sweet Cherry

- 1 Skinned Black Plume

- 1 Cup Dr. Sebi's Stomach Calming Herbal Tea/ Cuachalate back powder,

- ¼ Coconut Water

Directions:

1. Flash 1 teaspoon of Raisin in warm water for 5 seconds and drain the water completely.

2. Rinse, cube Sweet Cherry and skinned black Plum

3. Get 1 cup of water boiled; put ¾ Dr. Sebi's Stomach Calming Herbal Tea for 10 – 15minutes.

4. If you are unable to get Dr. Sebi's Stomach Calming Herbal tea, you can alternatively, cook 1 teaspoon of powdered Cuachalate with 1 cup of water for 5 – 10 minutes, remove the extract and allow it to cool.

5. Pour all the ARPS items inside a blender and blend till you achieve a homogenous smoothie.

6. It is now okay, for you to enjoy the inevitable detox smoothie.

Nutrition: Calories: 150 Fat: 1.2 g Carbohydrates: 79 g Protein: 3.1 g

Nori Clove Smoothies (NCS)

Preparation time: 10 minutes

Cooking time: 0 minutes

Servings: 1

Ingredients:

- ¼ Cup Fresh Nori

- 1 Cup Cubed Banana

- 1 Teaspoon Diced Onion or ¼ Teaspoon Powdered Onion

- ½ Teaspoon Clove

- 1 Cup Dr. Sebi Energy Booster

- 1 Tablespoon Agave Syrup

Directions:

1. Rinse ANCS Items with clean water.

2. Finely chop the onion to take one teaspoon and cut fresh Nori

3. Boil 1½ teaspoon with 2 cups of water, remove the particle, allow to cool, measure 1 cup of the tea extract

4. Pour all the items inside a blender with the tea extract and blend to achieve homogenous smoothies.

5. Transfer into a clean cup and have a nice time with a lovely body detox and energizer.

Nutrition: Calories: 78 Fat: 2.3 g Carbohydrates: 5 g Protein: 6 g

Brazil Lettuce Smoothies (BLS)

Preparation time: 10 minutes

Cooking time: 0 minutes

Servings: 1

Ingredients:

- 1 Cup Raspberries

- ½ Handful Romaine Lettuce

- ½ Cup Homemade Walnut Milk

- 2 Brazil Nuts

- ½ Large Grape with Seed

- 1 Cup Soft jelly Coconut Water

- Date Sugar to Taste

Directions:

1. In a clean bowl rinse, the vegetable with clean water.

2. Chop the Romaine Lettuce and cubed Raspberries and add other items into the blender and blend to achieve homogenous smoothies.

3. Serve your delicious medicinal detox.

Nutrition: Calories: 168 Fat: 4.5 g Carbohydrates: 31.3 g Sugar: 19.2 g Protein: 3.6 g

OTHER DIABETIC RECIPES

Zucchini Cauliflower Fritters

Preparation Time: 10 minutes

Cooking Time: 15 minutes

Servings: 4

Ingredients:

- 2 medium zucchinis, grated and squeezed

- 3 cups cauliflower florets

- 1 tbsp. coconut oil

- 1/4 cup coconut flour

- 1/2 tsp. sea salt

Directions:

1. Steam cauliflower florets for 5 minutes.

2. Add cauliflower into the food processor and process until it looks like rice.

3. Add all ingredients except coconut oil to the large bowl and mix until well combined.

4. Make small round patties from the mixture and set aside.

5. Heat coconut oil in a pan over medium heat.

6. Place patties in a pan and cook for 3-4 minutes on each side.

7. Serve and enjoy.

Nutrition: Calories 68 Fat 3.8 g, Carbohydrates 7.8 g, Sugar 3.6 g, Protein 2.8 g, Cholesterol 0 mg

Roasted Chickpeas

Preparation Time: 10 minutes

Cooking Time: 30 minutes

Servings: 4

Ingredients:

- 15 oz. can chickpeas, drained, rinsed and pat dry

- 1/2 tsp. paprika

- 1 tbsp. olive oil

- 1/2 tsp. pepper

- 1/2 tsp. salt

Directions:

1. Preheat the oven to 450 F/ 232 C.

2. Spray a baking tray with cooking spray and set aside.

3. In a large bowl, toss chickpeas with olive oil, paprika, pepper, and salt.

4. Spread chickpeas on a prepared baking tray and roast in preheated oven for 25 minutes. Stir every 10 minutes.

5. Serve and enjoy.

Nutrition: Calories 158 Fat 4.8 g, Carbohydrates 24.4 g, Sugar 0 g, Protein 5.3 g, Cholesterol 0 mg

Peanut Butter Mousse

Preparation Time: 10 minutes

Cooking Time: 10 minutes

Servings: 2

Ingredients:

- 1 tbsp. peanut butter

- 1 tsp. vanilla extract

- 1 tsp. stevia

- 1/2 cup heavy cream

Directions:

1. Add all ingredients into the bowl and whisk until soft peak forms.

2. Spoon into the serving bowls and enjoy.

Nutrition: Calories 157 Fat 15.1 g, Carbohydrates 5.2 g, Sugar 3.6 g, Protein 2.6 g, Cholesterol 41 mg

Coffee Mousse

Preparation Time: 10 minutes

Cooking Time: 20 minutes

Servings: 8

Ingredients:

- 4 tbsp. brewed coffee

- 16 oz. cream cheese, softened

- 1/2 cup unsweetened almond milk

- 1 cup whipping cream

- 2 tsp. liquid stevia

Directions:

1. Add coffee and cream cheese in a blender and blend until smooth.

2. Add stevia, and milk and blend again until smooth.

3. Add cream and blend until thickened.

4. Pour into the serving glasses and place in the refrigerator.

5. Serve chilled and enjoy.

Nutrition: Calories 244 Fat 24.6 g, Carbohydrates 2.1 g, Sugar 0.1 g, Protein 4.7 g, Cholesterol 79 mg

Wild Rice and Black Lentils Bowl

Preparation time: 10 minutes

Cooking time: 50 minutes

Servings: 4

Ingredients:

- Wild rice

- 2 cups wild rice, uncooked

- 4 cups spring water

- ½ teaspoon salt

- 2 bay leaves

- Black lentils

- 2 cups black lentils, cooked

- 1 ¾ cups coconut milk, unsweetened

- 2 cups vegetable stock

- 1 teaspoon dried thyme

- 1 teaspoon dried paprika

- ½ of medium purple onion; peeled, sliced

- 1 tablespoon minced garlic

- 2 teaspoons creole seasoning

- 1 tablespoon coconut oil

- Plantains

- 3 large plantains, chopped into ¼-inch-thick pieces

- 3 tablespoons coconut oil

- Brussels sprouts

- 10 large brussels sprouts, quartered

- 2 tablespoons spring water

- 1 teaspoon sea salt

- ½ teaspoon ground black pepper

Directions:

1. Prepare the rice: take a medium pot, place it over medium-high heat, pour in water, and add bay leaves and salt.

2. Bring the water to a boil, then switch heat to medium, add rice, and then cook for 30–45 minutes or more until tender.

3. When done, discard the bay leaves from rice, drain if any water remains in the pot, remove it from heat, and fluff by using a fork. Set aside until needed.

4. While the rice boils, prepare lentils: take a large pot, place it over medium-high heat and when hot, add onion and cook for 5 minutes or until translucent.

5. Stir garlic into the onion, cook for 2 minutes until fragrant and golden, then add remaining **Ingredients** for the lentils and stir until mixed.

6. Bring the lentils to a boil, then switch heat to medium and simmer the lentils for 20 minutes until tender, covering the pot with a lid.

7. When done, remove the pot from heat and set aside until needed.

8. While rice and lentils simmer, prepare the plantains: chop them into ¼-inch-thick pieces.

9. Take a large skillet pan, place it over medium heat, add coconut oil and when it melts, add half of the plantain pieces and cook for 7–10 minutes per side or more until golden-brown.

10. When done, transfer browned plantains to a plate lined with paper towels and repeat with the remaining plantain pieces; set aside until needed.

11. Prepare the sprouts: return the skillet pan over medium heat, add more oil if needed, and then add brussels sprouts.

12. Toss the sprouts until coated with oil, and then let them cook for 3–4 minutes per side until brown.

13. Drizzle water over sprouts, cover the pan with the lid, and then cook for 3–5 minutes until steamed.

14. Season the sprouts with salt and black pepper, toss until mixed, and transfer sprouts to a plate.

15. Assemble the bowl: divide rice evenly among four bowls and then top with lentils, plantain pieces, and sprouts.

16. Serve immediately.

Nutrition: Calories: 333 Carbohydrates: 49.2 grams Fat: 10.7 grams Protein: 6.2 grams

Alkaline Spaghetti Squash Recipe

Preparation time: 10 minutes

Cooking time: 30 minutes

Servings: 4

Ingredients:

- 1 spaghetti squash

- Grapeseed oil

- Sea salt

- Cayenne powder (optional)

- Onion powder (optional)

Directions:

1. Preheat your oven to 375°f

2. Carefully chop off the ends of the squash and cut it in half.

3. Scoop out the seeds into a bowl.

4. Coat the squash with oil.

5. Season the squash and flip it over for the other side to get baked. When properly baked, the outside of the squash will be tender.

6. Allow the squash to cool off, then, use a fork to scrape the inside into a bowl.

7. Add seasoning to taste.

8. Dish your alkaline spaghetti squash!

Nutrition: Calories: 672 Carbohydrates: 65 grams Fat: 47 grams Protein: 12 grams